Living with a disability - Your journey ahead

Contents

Have you been going the wrong way?

Have you been looking at your disability as the part of you that should not be here?

But what if your disability could talk to you, what would be the message that it is trying to tell you?

If there is one thing that I would like you to gain from this book, it is to explore your disability in more detail and understand that it is a part of you that needs to be loved and accepted. This is such a hard pill to swallow; loving your disability, especially if it causes you extreme pain and suffering, physically and/or emotionally.

So, I hear you, I hear you because I am also of the masses of people that would send my disability nothing but hatred and panic, for thirty years, until it wore me down to a holt.

So, I ask you this: what is your worst case scenario with your disability?

Are you scared that no one will accept you?
Are you afraid that you must stop working?
Are you worried that your disability will become worse?

What's your worst case scenario?
Please write this down, as this is what we will explore.

As always, with all of the books that I write, I ask you to hold on to a journal and pen, as I take you on a journey; a journey of exploration and emotional reasoning, as you look at your disability under a magnifying glass.

From today onwards, I would like you to see your disability as an **energy force**; an energy that is a part of the whole 'you'.
We will look at this energy force and see just how powerful your thoughts are around it and how you have been treating it.

At the very least, you will discover what your relationship with your disability is, whether it is a healthy one or not.

Before we start, I would like to ask you, out of a score of 10, how do you feel about your disability? 1 being "I hate it and wish it wasn't here", 10 being "I fully love and accept it". Please write this score in your journal.

Shall we begin :-)

Not accepting

Accepting your disability is one of the wisest moves you will ever make.

The question is, are you ready to accept?

Instead of stating to yourself that you can't accept the way that you are, try asking yourself what it is that you now, can accept.

What part of this can you accept?

Please write this down and let's work with this.

From what you **can** accept, is this enough, or do you need to work on accepting more of your disability energy force?

As human beings, we all suffer various degrees of non-acceptance to whatever happens to us in life. What you are going through now is what everyone would go through if it happened to them and what millions already have gone through and are going through at this very moment too. Your suffering is a normal coping process to get through this. To make it a hell of a lot easier, try to accept that you are not alone throughout this, with your non-acceptance.

Whatever it is that you cannot accept, ask yourself if you are the only one in the world to have these non-acceptance feelings.

And the answer will always be “No".

The answer will always be that millions of others have the very same feelings too.

If you’re still holding onto the past and how your life used to be, before your energy force became a part of you; the past is not a part of your life now.

If you’re still in shock because of how debilitating this energy force is; it is part of a process that you will go through, before you become accepting of it. The quicker you deliberately accept, the quicker you will feel relief.

If you can’t support yourself because of this energy force; what options do you now have? There is a way, please don't give up.

If you’re lonely because of your disability energy force; loneliness will only manifest if you keep on feeding it. You need to be a warrior of inner peace and strength and this book will show you how.

If you feel lost because of this part of you that is now sticking around; you can find your way back if you ask for help.

If there is a hole in your life now, because of your disability; you can and will feel whole again.

If this time is a dark place for you as a result of your unwanted energy force; there is always light at the end of the tunnel, once you have passed through.

We now know what you can accept within this disability energy force.

If you feel ready, write down what you cannot accept.

For example - My own past experiences from Hemiplegic migraine:

I cannot accept the frequency of attacks I am having

I cannot accept the memory loss and limb weakness

I cannot accept the panic and racing thoughts

I cannot accept persistent ocular aura for weeks/months at a time

I cannot accept that I have a disability

I cannot accept that it is a part of me

I cannot accept it, full stop!

Please write down your list - what are you not accepting?

____

If you take all humans out of the world, what would you have?

A motionless world!

If you take all humans out of the world apart from yourself what would you have?

No-one to compare with, nothing to relate to.

If you take away the world, what would you have?

Nothing to hold on to.

If you made the world too small what would you have?

No space to explore your options.

If you didn't accept that some of the people around you may leave your life what would happen?

You would be forever in denial.

Does this mean anything to you, or do you think I am just jabbering on about people and the world?

Maybe I am....

What I am trying to say is, that, no matter what has happened, no matter what you have been through or are still going through, no matter what disability energy force you are holding, you will always be a part of the world, going through what others go through, until the day that you pass away. There will still be people in your life and the world and others will still be here for you.

If you can't accept what is, accept that you are not alone in this non- acceptance world and accept that you are still alive, breathing and eating with other people.

When you are in the non-accepting mindset, just as all your fellow humans are, you are slowing down your life, you are no longer going with the flow and you are resisting any options that you now have.

Looking deeper into this, is the reason for your non-acceptance due to SHOCK, is the reason LOSS or is the reason YOU?

Shock is a process that we go through in order to adjust to the truth. Loss is losing that working part of you, to disability and adjusting to a different way of life without. If the reason you cannot accept after shock and loss is YOU then look at you, look at your life, look at who's in it, look at what you have and what you want, where you feel you are going, who you want to stay with you, take a deep look at you and ask yourself:

“Am I not accepting what is now, because of me and my life now”

If it is you, you are changeable.

Only you can make yourself truly happy, if you're not happy with you and your life, how can you expect it from anything or anyone else? How can you expect anyone else to give you what you should lovingly give to yourself? Use this time to assess what you have and where you want to be and let go of the memory that is causing you this feeling of non-acceptance. Fill your time with different things and come into another cycle of life. We call this cycle 'The warrior cycle'.

My thoughts are with you and I look forward to your acceptance. One day, it will come to you and this day will bring you peace.

And from inner peace - glows your **whole** energy force.

Fear

Please don't be afraid of fear, it is something that you've made up from all the thoughts that you've had about your disability, and rightfully so, when things become too hard to manage. But the fear that you feel will not stop your disability, it will not heal you; in fact, it will add to the suffering that you are going through. Although fear is very real to you and I, it is also a feeling that has manifested into physical symptoms. To put it another way, we can talk ourselves into any feeling if practiced, let's say, sadness. We can convince ourselves that we are sad and practice sad thoughts until we magnify our sadness. Fear is no different; it is the emotion that you have magnified into real symptoms that then become out of control.

So, fear cannot hurt you. YOU however, can hurt 'you' and when you feel intense prolonged fear you are doing just that. You are hurting yourself. Your fearful thoughts are creating behaviours within your body that give fear a physical life form, such as chest pain or panic attacks. No one else is responsible for this but your thoughts from your dear old mind. As I sit here writing this, please believe me when I say that I am still practicing manifesting calmness when all I want to do is manifest fear. I am the world's worst human at staying calm, when panic arrives. Yet, my mind knows the drill, it knows what I need to do, to get the right outcome. It is a lifelong lesson, one that anyone with a disability will need to master, in order to have a more fulfilling life. I am on the first steps to mastering fear. I do this by sending the source of the problem, my unwavering love.

Here's my example.

I was diagnosed with hemiplegic migraines at aged 16. Symptoms mimic that of a stroke and this disability has been my biggest and most awful part of my life. It is now thirty years later and throughout my experiences with this type of migraine, I have had more panic attacks than I care to remember. I've tried every medication with no results, have had a nervous breakdown from continuous panic and spent countless amounts of money on private specialists and holistic therapies to try and rid this energy force, this disability.

But the one symptom that has caused me the most turmoil, has been the aura symptom. My specific aura is visual disturbance (ocular aura). Whist a migraine attack is underway, my vision is lost, up to seventy percent and on most occasions, I have memory loss and cannot remember my name or how to get home. Once the attack is over, my vision doesn't fully come back to normal for days, months and sometimes, on rare occasions, a whole year at a time. This isn't the problem; the real problem is that the visual disturbance tells my brain that I am going to have another migraine attack, 24/7, as aura is everywhere, I look and should only happen during a migraine attack. So, wherever I go, I have spent thirty years on high alert and anxiety, "can I get through a day at work without an attack", "What if I have an attack now, Infront of all these people", and so on.

The panic that is manifested from the symptom (aura), is far worse than the actual symptom and it has taken me many years to retrain my brain to LOVE aura and this is what I have named my energy force - Aura.

When she's around (most of the time) I allow her to reside within me until she wants to leave, I tell her I love her, as she is a part of myself, a part of me that I need to accept; that I must accept as there is no other way to inner peace.

Which brings me back to yourself.

If you can master your panic and hatred, you are the master of your own mind.

I want to show you how.

If your mind is on your side, you can achieve anything, including inner peace and happiness.

So, just to recap, your feelings of fear are an indication that you need to change your thoughts/direction/process, as what you are thinking is not working well for you.

Prolonged fearful thoughts are like having a virus on a PC. They will manifest into bigger fearful thoughts, more fearful thoughts, more fearful behaviours and habits which may form panic, despair, depression, panic attacks and so on. It's hard enough to have a disability, please don't make it worse for yourself by feeding it with fear.

If it has already gone this far, you can still clear your PC. It's never too late, but it is a big job and awareness is the key to a healthy PC.

As hard as it is for you to stop fear, if you want to stop it then you need to start at the beginning.

What symptoms are you struggling with?

Please write them down.

This may seem like an obvious thing to observe here, but it seems that you're struggling to control the negative feelings from your symptoms, so it's best to start with the thought.

Ask yourself:

"What is it that I struggle with from this symptom?"

For example:

No job security = I'm afraid that I won't be able to hold my job down if these symptoms persist.

No pain threshold = I'm afraid I'm at my pain threshold and can't take anymore.

What negative emotions do you feel?

Now ask yourself:

Do you love yourself enough to help yourself find a solution?

And do you think that reacting to these symptoms negatively, will bring you closer to helping yourself?

So, we need to put loving thoughts into your mind instead.

I know it's easier said than done, so here's where the next step will help you.

When you feel the negative emotion, turn it inside out.

Literally!

When you are going through the fear emotion, turn the thought that gave birth to fear, inside out.

Example

Fear of losing your job due to symptoms = Sending my symptoms a big hug and lots of love, for I do not know the outcome and only love and kindness, to my symptoms, will help my outcome. With my mind on my side, I can get through anything.

NO ONE CAN TELL YOU THAT YOU ARE SAFE WITH YOUR DISABILITY AND WILL ALWAYS HAVE A JOB, A HOME AND FOOD ON THE TABLE. BUT THE JOURNEY THROUGHOUT YOUR LIFE IS MUCH MORE IMPORTANT THAN ANY OUTCOME. AND YOUR JOURNEY MUST START AND FINISH WITH INNER PEACE - NO MATTER WHAT YOUR OUTCOME.

Your thoughts are what make fear become real. Whether you fear something or not makes no difference to what will happen in your life, so you may as well love those symptoms instead of hating them.

Thought = fear = negative outcome

Thought = love = positive outcome

Turn the thought inside out and on its way out.

FEAR is a false emotion arising into your reality.

So, you can go the wrong way, down the fear and hatred road, until you reach your limit. Or, you can break through this and start going the way of love and self-compassion, of accepting and allowing your symptoms to stay however long they want, as this isn't a choice that you have. Your symptoms have a right to reside within you as part of your disability energy force. To try separate 'you' from this force, is unrealistic and impossible.

The choice that you do have, is to love or hate that part of you that wants to fit in and be loved.

By loving your disability, you are loving yourself; that part of yourself that has longed for your acceptance.

Your vision and reality

Are you waiting and expecting a disability free body and mind? Is this realistic? Wanting to be a different person to what you truly are, is all a part of the non-acceptance thought process. Instead, accept your reality and let us work on learning to love it instead. I know that this isn't what you want to hear; you want the magic wand, the fairy tale ending. But life isn't serving you that; life is serving you a much bigger teaching than the norm; it is serving you the teaching of a love that only the wisest people can obtain. To love what you want to hate is a truly remarkable and noble lesson that will bring many benefits to your life. Mainly, it will put you back in sync with your life, as you are no longer resisting against the grain, you are flowing down stream, allowing and loving what you once may have hated. So, your vision should always match your reality. If your disability energy force is here to stay, your vision should only be, to love and accept it as it is, because it is a part of you.

It is time - time to love

It's time to ask your energy force for forgiveness.
Time to make a fresh start.
Time to change your whole programming around your disability.
Time to reinvent yourself.
Time to make a pact with yourself.
Time to promise always, to love, never to hate.
Time show it that you can change and be the better version of yourself.
Time to accommodate this energy force.
Time to treat it as if it belongs.
Time to always respect and give it its' rightful place in your mind and body.
Time to stop fighting it.
Time to reach new heights.
It is time to start your next cycle of life. We call this cycle, 'The Warrior'

If your disability energy force could talk

One of the biggest teachings to gain from your inner work with a disability, is to ask your energy force:

"How have I been treating you?"

Let's write it down. This may feel uncomfortable for you, now that you know that your disability is you, as all those intense and negative emotions that have come from you, have come back to you.

"How have you been treating your disability energy force up to this point in your life?"

Please write your answers down.

When I answered this question, it was pure hatred, panic and like it didn't belong to be. I would reject it 100% and held a constant vision of life without this disability energy force, without Aura.

With your answer to this question, how do you feel about what you've written? Do you still feel this way or are you starting to see now, that any negativity that you projected upon it was ultimately projected onto yourself?

If you hate your disability, you are hating yourself.
If you panic about your disability, you are sending panic to yourself.

When I write it this way, it seems so easy to grasp, yet, for thirty years, I did not grasp this; I thought that by hating and panicking about it, it would somehow make things better and I would get better; like some sort of ritual management where practicing panicking daily, would mean that I could get through the day easier.

Me and my dysfunctional mind!

The answer that you have written is so important to you, it shows you what your whole being has had to endure this whole time.

I want you to feel remorse for any negativity that you have in your answer. Feeling remorse is the first step into awareness of what you have been doing to your beautiful self.

You don't deserve anything but pure positive thoughts to yourself.

Like an alcoholic that doesn't see a problem drinking two bottles of wine each night. Yet she has liver damage, arthritis and depression. Her alcohol intake is mistaken for a moment of release, pleasure and coping; yet, it is the drinking that is causing the problems in the first place.

We are no different. We feed disability with hatred and disbelief every single day, we throw our negativity towards ourselves, about ourselves (our disability) and as a result, we become mentally and physically worse.

If you feed a cat a plant based diet only, that cat will become ill as it needs meat to survive. If you feed your disability nothing but abuse, mentally, verbally or physically, the body and mind that is attached to that disability energy force, will become corrupt, dysfunctional and ill.

Today, your answer has shown you the path that you have been going down. I have a feeling (as this book has come to you) that it's the wrong path.

Today, feel remorse for the old path that you have trodden.

Forgive yourself.

From tomorrow, your new path starts.

From tomorrow, you are no longer like the alcoholic; from tomorrow you are on full detox!

This is your chance to love what needs loving.

All bark and no bite

Please divide those symptoms that you have from your energy force, into two divisions. Symptoms that are life-threatening and symptoms that are not.

With this rule, we must be black and white in our thinking here, as there are so many symptoms that fit into the 'grey' area. But let's stick to the plan.

You may have life-threatening symptoms and non-life-threatening symptoms. Please write down, under two headings, the life-threatening and non-life-threatening symptoms that you have.

Non-life-threatening symptoms - This means that whenever you get a symptom, no matter how painful and/or debilitating it is, you MUST tell your energy force that you are on its' side, that you love it and want to help it to feel safe. Talk to your energy force and feed it with love as this is the most spiritual practice that you can give to yourself. Your life lesson is so big and great. Your life lesson is to allow your disability to be a teacher of peace or a teacher of fear. Please choose peace and feed it with love. The outcome of loving your energy force will be:

Better mental health
Acceptance
Wise mindset
More capability
More independence
More confidence

No inner conflict
Living in sync with your universe
Reaching new spiritual practices
Building inner resilience
No longer playing the victim
A different perspective
A new life

The list goes on.
When love is in your heart, you open like a flower, to all possibilities; but mainly, that part of yourself that was always longing for your love, will now feel complete, regardless of your symptoms.

Life-threatening symptoms - This means that whenever you get a symptom, no matter how painful and/or debilitating it is, you MUST tell your energy force that you are on its' side, that you love it and want to help it to feel safe. Talk to your energy force and feed it with love as this is the most spiritual practice that you can give to yourself. Your life lesson is so big and great. Your life lesson is to allow your disability to be a teacher of peace or a teacher of fear. Please choose peace and feed it with love.

The outcome of loving your energy force will be:

Better mental health
Acceptance
Wise mindset
More capability

More independence
More confidence
No inner conflict
Living in sync with your universe
Reaching new spiritual practices
Building inner resilience
No longer playing the victim
A different perspective
A new life

The list goes on.

When love is in your heart, you open like a flower, to all possibilities; but mainly, that part of yourself that was always longing for your love, will now feel complete, regardless of your symptoms.

As you can see, both life-threatening and non-life-threatening, have the same answer, because no matter how hard it gets, no matter how intense your disability energy force is, it needs your compassion and love. Not because it's the easy route and seems like a pointless exercise that won't heal you. No. It needs your love because the other way will bring you down, hold you back, make you feel pointless and worthless every single day and take you far, far away from the feeling of being at home in your heart.

We must do the right thing for ourselves and start to love.

Get your mind on your side and the world will seem possible once more.

Give your disability a name

It's yours, it deserves a name, it deserves to be heard. What would you like to call it? Naming your energy force will help you to establish a good relationship with it, as you are pinpointing specifically to it, through it's given name.

As you know, Aura is what I call my energy force. Aura is a pretty name I think, and I know now that she is not life-threatening, although a very grey area, but never life-threatening. Yet. She won't hurt me; she just wants to stay until she leaves. The real problem wasn't Aura, it was my constant reaction of fear to her. I found her so debilitating and she was a great teacher of fear, until I cracked and reached the bottom, where I could no longer be a student of fear. That's when I learnt that she can also teach me to love. I am still learning to love Aura, I try with all my might, to welcome Aura and migraine and make her comfortable for the duration. I now accept her and react with compassion, knowing that Aura is in fact myself; we were never separate. She can cause me to break down or she can teach me what real calmness is; by how I react. She can be my biggest fear or my greatest teacher of how to be calm through an Aura storm.

Make friends with your symptoms so that at least your mental health is not knocked too much. This doesn't mean give up trying to heal but to make friends with your symptoms while on your healing journey path.

Please give your energy force a name

Just two choices

You only have two choices; to love it or hate it and that is it.

Imagine there are two wolves, fighting to win each other; one wolf is full of hatred and fear, the other is full of love and compassion. Which wolf will win depends only on the one that you feed. Feed your wolf with hatred and you shall become all things 'hatred'; feed your wolf with love and you shall become all things 'love'.

Where there is fear, there is an opportunity for love and growth.

Your job is to replace your fear and hatred wolf with your love and peace wolf. This is an extremely hard job for you, but remember, those especially hard jobs eventually become easier and easier with practice.
You have been creating the same habits of fear and hate; now you must create new healthier habits of love, compassion and peace, for doing this will retrain your mind to be on your side - I repeat throughout the book - you can get through anything when your mind is in your side.

Summarising your energy

I'd like you to finish off the following sentences, write it down and then read it back to yourself so that you understand yourself a little better.

My biggest difficulty with my disability, is………This is causing me to feel…….I struggle to handle my emotions because……….My biggest physical problems are……… and my biggest mental health problems are………. As a result, I do less of……… and more of……… and cannot get the balance between………and……..This disability is causing me to……… As a result.

And now read it back to yourself to see how you feel about your answers. I hope it brings some insight to your feelings, around your energy force and I want this book to reach out to you and support you in every way possible, that is within my reach for you.

I also want to say, at this point, I don't know exactly what you are going through, but I do know what the emotional pain feels like, when your life stops and everything revolves around your disability. I know it can be exhausting; I know it can make you feel suicidal, depressed, anxious and all sorts of intense and dark feelings. I can only write this because of the very dark times I have been through with Aura. But we must remember that we always come out of the other side; stronger, wiser, braver. We are given a huge life difficulty; but in every difficulty, there is a great big gift wrapped inside; the gift of being a warrior of peace through pain and suffering.

Find that gift and you find one of life's biggest secrets.

Let that gift be a teacher of peace and love, through suffering, not a teacher of fear and hatred through suffering.

Time to stop

Please write all the things you need to stop doing.

For example:

I need to stop hating Aura
I need to stop isolating myself
I need to stop focusing all my energy onto Aura
I need to stop…

I need to stop……………………………………

And now, put a date next to each thing written. A date that you want to reach this goal.

For example:

I need to stop hating Aura, by Jan 2020.
I need to stop isolating myself by March 2020.
And so on.

Time to start

Please write all the things you need to start doing.

For example:

I need to start being braver and going out more regardless of the attacks.

I need to start meditating each day
I need to own Aura and not be embarrassed if I have an attack in front of others

I need to start…………………………………………

And put a date next to each thing written.

Letting go

Write all the things you need to let go of.

For example:

I need to let go of the expectation that I will one day lose this disability.
I need to let go of wanting my body to be reliable for work on a constant basis
I need to let go of fear and panic

I need to let go of…………

And again, please write the dates of when you would like to let go by.

For example:

I will let go of the expectation that I will lose this disability - immediately.
I will let go of the expectation that my body is reliable for work on a constant basis - by the end of this week.

Love what you can

Write all the things you need to love about your energy force.

For example:

I need to love Aura and her visual disturbances because she is a part of me.
I need to love migraine attacks because they are a part of me.
I need to love and accept bed rest when I am unable to do anything else.

(please notice how I am stating that I love Aura, migraines etc, because they are a part of myself. I am NOT stating that I love having aura, migraine attacks etc, as this would send the message to myself that I love having all these debilitating symptoms. I am simply loving what is a part of me, not asking for more of it, but accepting it is here, because it is a part of myself).

To make it easier for yourself, simply state:

"I love you disability, because you are a part of me".

This ensures that you are giving your mind the correct message; to love what is, nothing more, just to love what is.

Please write what you need to love.

I need to love……………………………………………

And now, write the dates next to each thing written.

Now you have a plan.

Going with the flow

Like the river that flows downstream, not against it, just along with the current; even when there are storms and waterfalls, rocks and boulders, the river never ever goes against the current. It would be impossible to even try.

So why do we? Why do we fight our energy force with hatred and panic; why do we punish ourselves further when we are already suffering enough? You are the stream; your disability is the current; don't fight it! Go with it and allow it to pass through you, no matter what storms and waterfalls lie ahead.

Boomerang projecting

I've spoken briefly about this earlier in the book, so apologies if I am repeating myself, but whatever emotion you feel, is the emotion that is projected back onto yourself. Your emotions are like a boomerang; let's say you feel happy and you are giving out happy vibes. To give out happy vibes, you must also experience them back. This may seem like everyone knows this but if we look closer, what we don't see is that those negative emotions that we feel about our disability, those emotions bounce right on back to us.

Like a mirror, you look and see an image and decide whether you like what you see. You decide from your disability, what you want to feel about it and project that emotion out, and then, that emotion comes back inside of your mind and you think 'hey, I don't like this emotion, how do I stop it'. You can only stop it by stopping the original thought about how you feel about your disability. Instead of looking at your energy force and feeling sad, look at your energy force and feel an emotion that is easier to handle than sad, such as acceptance or to tolerate it today.

'Just for today'. In order to retrain the brain to think like this, you must control your thoughts and your reaction to your symptoms.

Here's my example:

Having a hemiplegic migraine attack - My initial thought was panic. After around three seconds, I became aware that I was panicking, (projection boomeranging) and changed the thought to "Ah, hello Aura, welcome. I allow you to reside here, I love you because you are a part of me".

The outcome is that the emotion that I gave out was peace and in return I received peace back.

That makes me a warrior of peace

This is not an easy process; what I am asking of you is to change your whole thought process around your energy force; I am asking you to become a warrior of peace. In fact, I am begging you to become a warrior of peace because I want you to protect your mental health. If there is nothing that we can do about our disability, we must accept it, we must love it as part of ourselves, we must give ourselves that break and go with the current; go with the flow.

Since loving Aura, there has been a huge shift in my mindset, like the missing jigsaw piece that I could never find, that would help me to love myself fully. There is no longer any war internally and when I become afraid that Aura will stop me from holding a job down and surviving on my own, financially; I talk to her, I tell her "it's gonna be ok, and no matter what happens in my life and around work, I will always love Aura, I will always accept her; because to do anything else is not only a waste of my energy, it causes ill mental health that cripples me more than Aura does. And let's not forget that ill mental health is another disability - I call my anxiety, Anna. and when she visits I affirm to her that she is safe, 100 times every day.

So, my friend, I am asking you to become a 'warrior of peace' and protect yourself from negative boomerang projecting.

Are you with me?

Are you with me?

Are you with me!!!!!!!!!!

I hope to hell you said yesssss!! I was shouting as I wrote that. I want the best life for you and to get that, you MUST pledge to be a warrior of peace, to react with love and peace as soon as you want to react with panic or hatred.

Now, please write in your journal "I am a warrior of peace" sign and date it, because from today, you have agreed to myself and all the other readers that take the same pledge, that we are in this together, that we know how hugely difficult it is to be us and we choose to be warriors of peace.

You are enough

You are enough exactly as you are. Your circumstances are nothing to do with 'not feeling like you are enough', but they are a result of the boomerang thoughts that you have.

Just to set the record straight, there is not one person in this universe that is born without a soul. Our bodies may be different to each other's but fundamentally, we are all the same. The Queen still poops and the pope still picks his nose. And yes, we are all as worthy as each other; exactly the same worthiness is placed within each one of us, but what stops us from feeling worthy, are those boomerang thoughts. If you practiced stating the affirmation:

"I am worthy"

One thousand times every day, after several months you will feel more worthy; after one year you will feel worthier still as your boomerang thoughts are coming back to you and sending you worthy vibes.

What you put out, you get back - thoughts out, boomerang thoughts back.

At some point, you started the thought **"I am not worthy"** and so, the boomerang projection began.

In a relationship

The sooner you accept that you are in a relationship with your disability, the easier this will be. Treat your energy force how you would like to be treated yourself, because, as you know, it is you and you are in a relationship with that part of yourself.

Have you been the abusive partner that has verbally knocked your energy force to the ground? If this is true, it's never too late to be that nice partner, to make it up to your disability and ask for forgiveness - to be a **warrior of peace**.

I treated Aura terribly, but I made a fresh start and promised to love her like I would want to be loved myself. Your disability and you are together for life, so you need to show it some love and respect, to do anything different is disrespecting yourself.

Defining your life

Your disability does not destroy your life, it defines it. Even as I write this, it feels difficult to say and I know many of you will disagree. And, of course, I am not always right. But in most cases; it's the fear of what your disability is capable of at its worst case scenario, that destroys us and any hope and joy that we have. But as newly pledged warriors, with our minds on our side and a peaceful heart; with our disability we can become the defined warrior that we are; free from inner mental turmoil as, we embrace what storms come our way, allowing this energy force to define us in a healthier way rather than projecting ill mental health onto ourselves. Please don't think that your body has failed you; the opposite is true. Your body has pushed through a tremendous amount of suffering and pain; that is not failure, that is continued success. To keep on jumping those hurdles and moving forwards is success in its highest and truest form.

Positive self-talk - Defining your life always starts at the beginning, with positive self-talk. Please write in your journal, a typical day, of getting up and how you talk to yourself around your disability. For example:

"I hope I don't have an attack today, can I get through a day without an attack, my eyes are fucked, I'm panicking so much about my vision, this isn't normal, there's something seriously wrong with me, everything looks slanted, I don't feel connected to my body, I can't handle a whole day of this, what time is it,

I need to get ready quickly, I'm late, why am I always late. I need to stop spending money and start to be stricter on my expenditure, I can do better than this, what if I lose my job, how will I pay off my debt". Wish I lived alone, I could be as ill as I like if I was alone. It's so hard to pretend to be well when I'm dying inside".

You get the picture?

And yes, these are real thoughts from my past. It would be VERY easy for me to slip back into them like an old pair of pyjamas, but those pyjamas didn't keep me peacefully warm. I had to fight for peace and so do you, until your mind is reprogrammed, until you can peacefully get on with your day, disability and all.

Please write down a typical day's monologue.

Now, I'd like you to read through it and ask yourself if it is full of peace?

More than likely, it won't be. You are now aware of your daily self-talk. Does it look healthy to you?
What would you like to change?
Please write down what you would change.

For example: "If I have an attack today, I'll be fine, I can I get through an attack peacefully if I focus on reciting peaceful thoughts such as "I love you Aura, do your thing". My visual disturbance is being imaginative, I'm choosing peace about my vision, this vision isn't the norm but it will pass and my job is to stay peaceful throughout. Aura is really trying to challenge me today, she is challenging me to choose peace or panic, I will choose peace. My world looks slanted and this is quite cool as I know it's temporary. I don't feel connected to my body but I know that I am connected and I just need to put my hand on my heart, look in the mirror and tell Aura I love her as she is me. A whole day of this will be hard but it's never impossible. What time is it, I need to get ready, I'm late but I will not rush. I will get up earlier tomorrow and focus on getting there earlier. I need to stop spending money and start to be stricter on my expenditure, I can do this, I just need a plan. If I lose my job, I will find a way to pay off my debt". Wish I lived alone, I could be as ill as I like if I was alone. It's so hard to pretend to be well when I'm dying inside but also it helps be to push myself and fake it until I make it back to good health".

Same problems, different monologue.

Practice your **warrior of peace** stance and re-write what you can change.

The secret is to stay calm and not react but to think of well thought out responses. This takes practice as you are retraining the brain and the brain is very stubborn. If, like me, you've had a lifetime of feeding your disability with hatred and panic, guess what, it will take you a while to retrain the brain to peace and love.

But it is NEVER EVER impossible, so start now and give yourself time. You must work it, like you're at the mind gym, working out for a peaceful mind.

This means watching all the thoughts that come from your mind and out of your mouth; stopping those negative thoughts and replacing them with peace and love. Practicing until you master this. That's the peace warrior within you!

Those triggers

Does your disability have triggers? In most cases, it will. Those triggers are that part of yourself, stating to you "hey, I don't like this, please stop". If you are ignoring your triggers, you are ignoring yourself and, in some cases, this is self-abuse.

The person with liver damage, drinking large quantities of alcohol and making himself ill.
The person with IBS that eats food she shouldn't and becomes very ill the next day.
The Person with lupus that does intense cardio workouts, four days a week and feels burnt out at the weekends.
The person with heart disease that smokes forty cigarettes a day and can't walk far.

What are your triggers? Are you self-abusing or do you listen to your energy force and stay away from your triggers?

Please write down what your triggers are.

And next to each trigger, write down whether you are abusing your body or not.

What are you willing to give up for your energy force?

The answer should be 'whatever it takes to be the best version of myself possible'.

So, if giving up alcohol is needed, in order to heal liver damage, it's a no brainer. Of course, I understand addiction, but you must also understand self-abuse and ask yourself 'what am I going to do about it'. Do nothing and your disability will grow until it becomes too big to handle.

What's meaningful in my life

Imagine life free from pain and/or emotional turmoil. Imagine for a moment, life without your disability energy force.

What would make life meaningful for you if you could do anything and be anywhere?

Please write it down before you read on.

What makes my life meaningful is………?

And now add your energy force back.

And rewrite your list

What makes my life meaningful is……….?

In most cases, when I ran a peer support group on this topic, the outcome was that the list was very similar.

Some examples that were the same with and without disability are:
Travel
Family
Art
Colour
Cats
People
Love
Creating

Photography
Nature
Stillness

Most of the group had at least three of the same things on their list, living with disability as they did, living without. What this means is your disability shouldn't be stopping you from what is meaningful to you.

What is meaningful is what counts. Please don't give up on what matters to you the most.

The perfect host

Imagine now, a friend has come to stay. You've prepared the perfect space to be in. Soft cushions, warm hearty drinks, comfortable clothing and bedding for them, ample light, a brilliant view and lots of love, laughter and deep, meaningful conversations. Your friend stays the whole weekend and leaves you feeling lifted and content.

That friend is your disability; and you, as the warrior of peace, need to be the perfect host while it stays. Always giving yourself the above as much as possible and never anything less.

This is a true warrior's heart.

The victim

We can spend our whole lives playing the victim.

"Why me"
"No one understands how bad this is"
"No one fucking listens to me"
"No one cares"
"I'm so alone"
"I can't take it anymore"
"I want to die"
"I wish I wasn't here"
"I'm a burden to everyone"
"No one wants to hear my continuous problems"

These are real thoughts that are usually brought about because your threshold has reached its' limit. Your mind has had enough and as a result, you've fallen into the 'self-pity pit'. Hey, we've all been there, I'm no different. But reaching within and practicing the warrior of peace, will help you to get out of that pit and start to accept and work with what you've got, whether that's ten fingers or none.

If you were born with your disability, you won't know how it feels to be any different, but you may have a strong urge to be disability free as you grow and see others around you, looking like they are having a good life. And so, you fall into the victim pit. Or, you may have become disabled in some way, as you have grown, experiencing life before and after your energy force came to you. And so, you want what you used to have, also falling into the victim pit.

Both are extremely hard to deal with and being in the pit magnifies this hardship by 100%. That's 100% harder than it could be. Ok, I'm making that bit up, but believe me, if you're in the pit today, your saviour is the warrior of peace. Practicing the thoughts and changing them, retraining the mind until you eventually surface from the pit. Once you're out of the pit, you'll work extra hard at the mind gym, to never fall into that excruciating pit again. Believe me, I'm at the mind gym daily!

Being in the victim pit, you are punishing yourself and putting all the blame on yourself when in fact, it is no-one's fault. No matter how you give birth to this energy force, it came to you as truth, pure truth of what is. And your job is to be a good host, not to punish, blame and self-sabotage, in a bid to be free of it. It's a pointless waste of time being in the pit but sometimes, I feel, a part of the process before you get to become a peace warrior. So, if you are in the pit today, know that tomorrow is brighter. Know that millions have been there, and the only way out is at the mind gym. By the way, the mind gym is a free subscription, so you should really take it.

Speaking directly

If we speak directly to our energy force and address it with the respect it deserves, in turn, you are sending love to yourself. Don't worry, your brain likes you to see your energy force as something you are having a relationship with because the brain needs to see and feel things in order to comply. So, having a name for your energy force, helps your brain to address it specifically. Being a good host to it, helps your brain to feel safe with it, showing it peace, trains your brain to erase bad habits. Even though you are all one big brain, there are parts of your brain for this and that, such as your ego and subconsciousness. So, there is a part of your brain that likes you to manage it and up until now, you may have let your brain go haywire, not managing it at all and ending up in the pit.

We are here to manage your brain and we do this by naming your disability first and managing it with love and peace. We also ask our disability for forgiveness from all past hatred. The brain will then associate that it is separate to disability and want to accommodate it with your new instructions.

Managing for power and confidence

The best way to manage your energy force is to be still and listen to what it needs. Sit in a chair with a cup of tea and stare at the walls for one hour. Keep your journal with you for any ideas that spring to mind. Do everything slowly so that your body gets used to calmness and keep asking your energy force "what can I do for you, what do you need".

Largest and hardest falls

It's not enough for us to accept our energy force at its smallest; we must also accept it at its' largest and hardest falls. To do this, we must make friends with the scariest of our symptoms. Those symptoms that want to send us into panic mode and push us to our threshold. By letting go of how you want your body to be and love it for what it is. Let go of the expectation you have and what you want and allow your body and mind to be what it is. Let go of the vision that you have and accept the reality that is. Acceptance of your disability at its worst is when your whole world feels like it's falling down and everything is falling apart and you sink to the bottom, knowing that the only way from here, is up and into a new world of accepting and learning to live with your disability in a healthy and more peaceful way. This is a painful process but once you reach this point, you know you are healing your mind.

How to start loving

Start with the affirmation " I love you energy force (name), I welcome you to pass through my home".

Start stating this affirmation at least thirty times per day, until your mind stats to realise that you are in management mode now and the old way is not the right way.

I love you because? - Please write in your journal, five reasons why you love your energy force. This may feel very difficult but there is always a silver lining.

For example:

I love you Aura, because you've pushed me to study the mind, I don't take things for granted, I appreciate the good times, You have shown me how to panic and how to stop panicking, choosing the later. I love you because you've made me be very careful what I put into my body.

I love you because……………..?

Say the 'Ho Oponopono' prayer EVERY morning, in front of the mirror.
An ancient Hawaiian practice for processing inner thoughts and helping you to understand yourself and grow.

Please memorise the following:

I'm sorry
Please forgive me
I love you
I thank you

That is the prayer. State this daily, as part of your daily routine.

Here's some examples:

I'm sorry - For putting you through such inner turmoil.
Please forgive me- for putting you through all those thoughts of panic and hatred.
I love you - Because you are amazing and a true hero for what you endure.
I thank you - for putting up with me for all these years and trying your very best for me.

I'm sorry - For the symptoms that you have right now
Please forgive me - If there is nothing that I can do to help.
I love you - and want you to know how much I want to help you through this.
I thank you - for accepting these symptoms and sending them love and peace.

I love this prayer because each day, I give myself a different message; a message that my body really needs to hear, in that moment.

Daily breath - Spend ten minutes each day, sitting quietly and breathing deeply. Long deep breaths for ten minutes to circulate your blood flow and get any negativity shifted. While you do this, think of ten reasons to be grateful.

Practice love - Practice your new mindset, put it to the test and ask your body to bring on your unwanted symptoms. And then send those symptoms an overwhelming amount of love in whichever way you feel. Words are the most powerful so tell your symptoms you are sorry for never cooperating and how much you love it for it is you. Treat it how you treat your loved ones and be EXTRA kind to it because, 'it' is 'you'.

Welcome your energy force like an old friend

Out of your control

You will never be able to control your energy force towards disappearance. What is out of our control is no longer a choice of ours to have. So why try to control something that cannot be controlled? You are a duo, like the weeds in a flower garden, like the volcano and its eruption of lava. You may not like what you have been given and it may cause pain and discomfort, but you live together. The weeds do not fight the earth. The lava does not attack its volcanic shell, it is the aftermath that causes us to react how we do. If you can learn to love your energy force, no matter what, the aftermath will be faced much easier, with a peaceful heart.

Own it - own your disability. It is yours. It is you.

Make peace not war.

Be excited to start your new life together, in harmony, as you love the part of your brain that you always loathed. A truly marvellous life lesson and huge shift in your thinking ways.

Love is the answer to all wars, inner and out.

Finding a support system

Every disability needs a support system. A tribe of people that are going through exactly what you are going through. Connect with those people as they will have more compassion for your symptoms than anyone else. Find a group near you or an on-line group.

Save that date

Think of a date in the future, that you want to be excited about, for example - Christmas. A date that you can focus on with happy thoughts, with your new mindset about your disability. And work towards that goal.

For example:

It's August, I want to have my new mindset in full flow by Christmas. I want to turn my life around and fully love Aura and whatever storms she brings. I want to be socialising more, travelling more and being free of doubt. I want to embrace an attack if and when it happens, even if I am out and I want to welcome Aura, daily, as she appears before me, as she does. By Christmas day, I will be in love with Aura and Aura will be in love with me. We will work together in harmony and I will greet her as an old friend. By Christmas day, my life will be full of courage and peace and I will make sure that I never miss a God damn thing due to panicking about Aura and whether I will get through events. Fuck it, I will live my life fully and embrace this life with Aura in it.

Amen sisters and brothers!

What is your future event and date?
Please write it down.

And write how peaceful and brave you want to be.

Lastly - I would like you to revisit how you feel about your disability. At the beginning of the book, you gave yourself a score.

And what is your score now?
Out of 10, how do you feel about your disability?
1 being "I hate it and wish it wasn't here", 10 being "I fully love and accept it". Please write this score in your journal.

If your score has shifted, even one point, it is worth reading and practicing self-love.

You are now a **'warrior of peace'**.

Your new life should ALWAYS hold peace in your heart.

I wish an overwhelming amount of love to you and your energy force and hope that you hold peace in your heart, always - Olivia.

Hemiplegic migraines, Addison's Disease, 5 different cancers, bone degeneration of back (4 surgeries, 2 fusions and pain stimulator) knee replacement, hip replacement, then had a dislocated hip, lung damage from 3 bouts of double pneumonia, 3 holes in my heart. I'm only 54 and have the spine of a 90 year old as my neurosurgeon has told me! What gets me through is to be your own best advocate along with your partner or family. I have treatment protocols from my Dr's - Shirlieann Texas

Justyna - UK. I have rheumatoid arthritis and Lupus, both autoimmune diseases. I am winning with lupus so far and I will share with you, how I've done this. My symptoms are whole day fatigue, unbelievable tiredness due to ongoing inflammation around the joints and low iron level. Most of the time I'm in huge pain all over my body, there are no breaks from it, in my case, it's mainly my arm, jaw, knees, feet, fingers, toes, hips and wrist, to the point you're not able to hold a mug, zip buttons or stand up, to walk, and do a simple tasks.

This disability effects the emotional and mental side too and sometimes I feel really depressed. What gets me through, in my case, no matter how down I get, I am always trying my best to move forward and not to stay stuck in this darkness.

I am determined to heal so much that I have found a breathing technique that has been life changing for me. I am so convinced that this technique works that I studied to be a holistic breath coach and have spent time on myself until I could see magnificent results. Each breathing session helps me to feel more energised due to an increase in oxygen. I am still on my healing journey but so glad I was introduced to this technique. I realise now that my path is to help others with inner healing and have created a website with more information - www.thrive3.co.uk

Susan - UK - I have very bad arthritis and have also had my bowels taken away. My symptoms are stiffness, swelling, restlessness, joint pain and having to use a bag on my stomach so that I can go to the toilet. What's hard for me is that I have no control over flatulence or when I defecate, sometimes it happens when I'm around people. No one knows this as the bag that is fitted to my stomach, isn't visible, but sometimes the flatulence makes noises into my bag and that embarrasses me. What gets me through is telling myself how luck I am to have a roof over my head, food in the cupboard, shoes on my feet and a warm bed each night. I may be in pain sometimes or embarrassed other times, but I'm still a lucky soul to have all the basic things that make me feel safe and content.

Hemiplegic migraine completely changed my life and career of a RN at the age of 35. I am now a stay at home mom, left unable to drive and needing help with my children. It paralyzes my left side with episodes, but the lasting cognitive effects of mental awareness and judgement have never gone away since my 1st attack. I have given up so much as most of you all do with a HM disease. My few mottos I have forced to live by are: "You may see me struggle from time to time, but you will NEVER see me give up" "adjust your lifestyle to find a way to live life to its fullest, not allowing the disability to not let you live" and "look for the positive in any darkened day because there is something positive always around you, you just have to be willing to look for it!" Good luck to all our warrior friends!
REBECCA...MI, USA

I'm a 39 year old former preschool teacher who has had Hemiplegic Migraines since age 6. In recent years I've acquired multiple complex chronic conditions that have led to being unable to work. Living with chronic illness is a daily struggle, with fatigue, loss of sense of self/purpose, and unpredictable symptom flares. It is important to self-advocate, keep close the people and things that bring you joy, and to take each day moment by moment. ~Sabrina Arana, Oregon, USA.

I have Bipolar Disorder and have been sectioned twice after having two psychosis episodes. My symptoms are extreme highs and lows. When I'm really low, I can't get out of bed, when I'm really high, I also hallucinate and have gone AWOL a few times, ending up in another country once and not knowing how I got there. I've got myself into a lot of trouble over the years. My saving grace is my medication. Without it, I'm unable to have a normal balanced life. The side effects from the meds are mainly that I have lost the ability to have intense feelings, for example, when I should be grieving for a loss, I struggle to feel that grief, or any feeling really. But this is a much better swap than life before medication, believe me. I nearly lost my kids to this disability. Now I can live and work again! - Tina London, 45, UK.

I'm 25 years old. I'm a Paramedic. I'm currently having to take time off from my job because of Hemiplegic Migraines. When I have an attack, it paralyzes the right side of my body, I can't talk, and sometimes it effects my vision. Due to the sporadic nature of HM I can't do my job, taking care of patients. I've had 2 helicopter rides to stroke centres, due to this disability. I'm currently seeking disability support. I keep my family close. I pray every day that I wake up headache free. Most people don't understand HM and "it's just a headache". My faith keeps me going and hope for medications that will fully control symptoms. - Michelle, AL, USA

Thank you to all of our brave warriors that have submitted these stories to us and continue to be a warrior of promoting inner peace.

Other books by Olivia Bowden @ frontdoorpublishing.com

- The Secret Guide A-Z self-help (150 topics of self-help)

- A pocket guide through heartache

- I hate the way I look

- Find yourself first - before choosing the right partner

- Billy be good - children's educational books

Resources - Wendy Francis - Creator of the concept 'energy force'
Ho'oponopono prayer: An ancient Hawaiian practice for forgiveness and reconciliation.

Made in the USA
Monee, IL
08 November 2026

67972909R00037